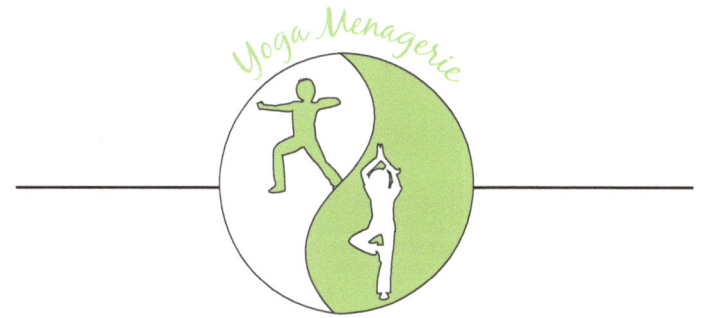

For My Children
Drake and Zoe;
May You Always Follow Your Flow

_____

Yoga Menagerie's
MUDRAS
RE'FLEX'IONS
Book Three

BY: VICTORIA FISHMAN
ILLUSTRATED BY: MORGAN KELLER

Mudra is pronounced "moo-drah." It is most often translated as "seal" or "lock." Mudras are symbolic gestures, primarily done with the hands. Sometimes mudras are described as "yoga for the hands." The language of gestures is able to convey more significance for the mind than just words alone can express.

You can practice mudras at any time and in any place. Mudras can be performed standing, sitting, lying down, being still or moving. It is important to remember to perform mudras with ease and relaxation. You shouldn't force the fingers or hold them in a position that is painful. You should always feel relaxed when doing mudras.

Mudras can be intensified by adding in breathing exercises and positive affirmations. Each Mudra in this book is titled with its Sanskrit names as well as an English translation. Place your fingers as shown in the picture and as described at the bottom of each page. Each mudra also comes with a rhyming verse to remind you what each mudra is used for and gives the mind something to focus on. Doing mudras and saying the verse helps to promote the mind-body connection.

When applying breathing techniques to the mudras you can focus on the pressure of the fingers in multiple ways. During both the inhale and the exhale you can focus on the sensation of the touching the fingers together. You can also release that tension during the exhale and apply pressure as you inhale. This can also be done in reverse by applying tension during the inhalation and releasing it during the exhalation. *The number of breaths and their duration during practice is relative and changeable to adapt to all skill levels. MUDRAS ARE FUN AND EASY TO DO. COME EXPLORE THE WOMDERFUL EXPERIENCE OF USING MUDRAS!

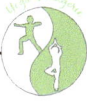

The Adventure Guide

MUDRAS BOOK (BOOK THREE)

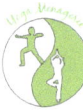

MUDRA IS PRONOUNCED "MOO-DRAH." IT IS MOST OFTEN TRANSLATED AS SEAL OR LOCK. MUDRAS ARE SYMBOLIC GESTURES, PRIMARILY DONE WITH THE HANDS.

26 Granting Wishes or Mercy – Varada Mudra

27 Confidence – Ahamkara Mudra

28 Balancing – Mahasirs Mudra

29 Stress Relief – Dwimukham Mudra

30 Calming – Chinmaya Mudra

31 Victory – Humkara Mudra

32 Peace – Bhu Mudra

33 Love – Purna Mudra

34 Relaxation – Matsya Maudra

35 Inner Strength – Brahma Mudra

36 Power/Fist – Mushti Mudra

37 Beak – Mukula Mudra

38 Air/Wind – Vayu Mudra

39 Sky /Emptiness – Shunya Mudra

40 Sun – Surya Mudra

41 Earth – Prithivi Mudra

42 Water – Varuna Mudra

43 Heart – Apan Vayu Mudra

44 Shell – Shankh Mudra

45 Thunderbolt – Vajra Mudra

46 Bird – Garuda Mudra

47 Bee – Bhramara Mudra

48 Elephant – Ganesha Mudra

49 Crocodile – Makara Mudra

50 Snake/Strength & Wisdom – Naga Mudra

MUDRAS

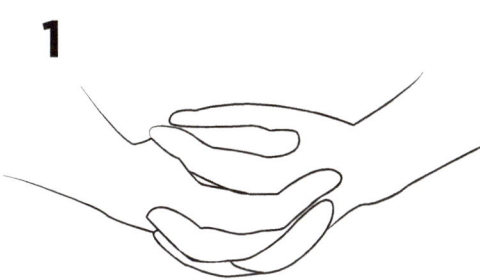

1

NEW BEGINNINGS
ORIGIN OF ALL THINGS GOOD
USHAS MUDRA

I am ready to experience something new;
Beginnings expand my point of view.

*Clasp your hands with your fingers laced
together. (Right thumb on top of the left)*

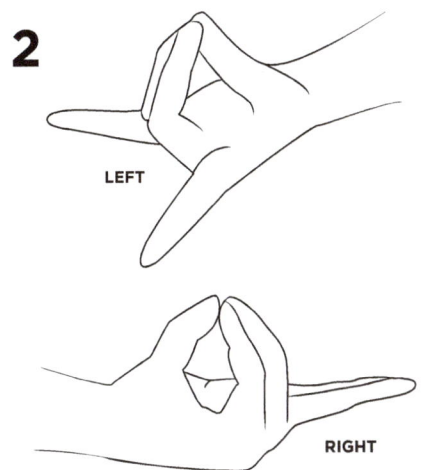

LEFT

RIGHT

2

RECEIVING AND LETTING GO
PUSHAN MUDRA

I receive the things that keep me on track;
And let go of the things that hold me back.

*Right hand – touch the tips of the thumb, index, and middle
fingers – extend the others
Left hand – Touch the tips of the thumb, middle and ring
finger – extend the others*

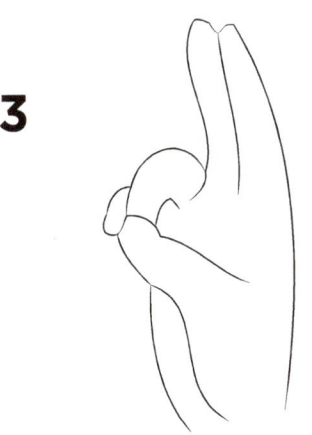

3

LIFE AND ENERGY
PRAN MUDRA

My inner strength and endurance see me through –
There is nothing I can't do.

*Touch the tips of the thumb, ring and pinky fingers –
extend the others*

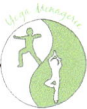

4

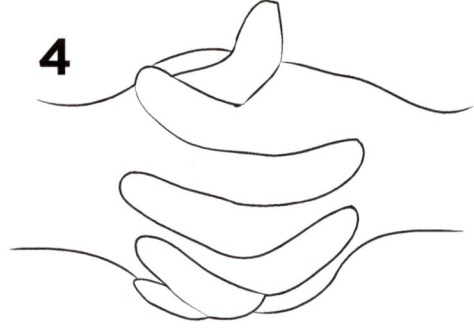

RELEASING
LINGA MUDRA

My powers of resistance are very strong;
Yet I can release the things that don't belong.

Clasp your hands – one thumb should remain up – circle it with the thumb and index finger of the other hand

5

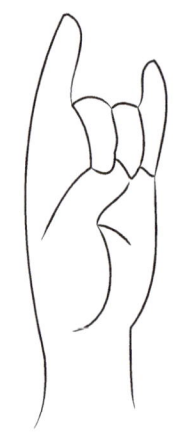

ENERGY
APAN MUDRA

I am balanced – I am serene;
I am moving forward, following my dreams.

Touch the tips of the thumb, middle and ring fingers together – extend the others

6

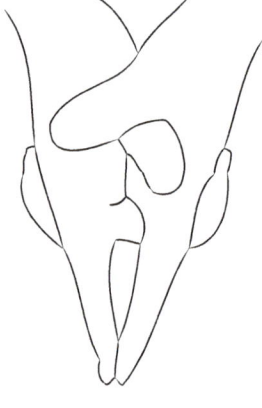

LETTING GO /POURING OUT
KSEPANA MUDRA

I pour out the things I must let go;
And let in the things that help me grow.

Clasp your hands together – extend the index fingers up and touch the together – cross the thumbs over each other (point fingers down)

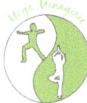

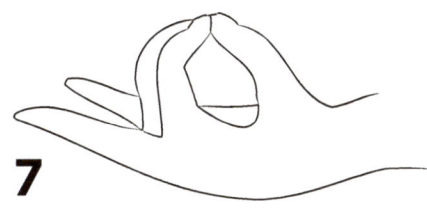

CENTERING
RUDRA MUDRA

I am centered – I am sure;
My strength comes from my inner core.

Touch the tips of the thumb, index and ring fingers together – extend the others

7

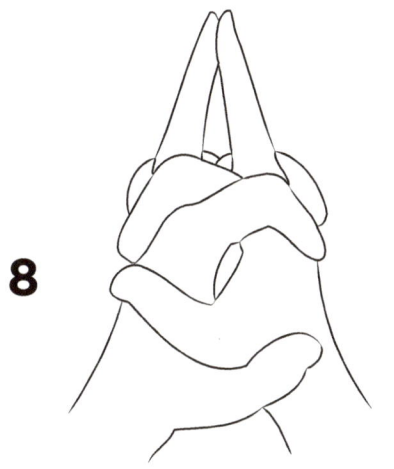

INNER HARMONY
MATANJI MUDRA

I am at peace – I can let things be;
I maintain inner harmony.

Clasp your hands together – extend the middle fingers up and touch them together

8

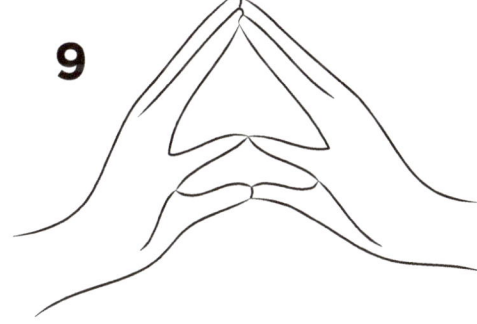

FOCUS
HAKINI MUDRA

I can concentrate and focus my mind;
I can remember ideas and keep my thoughts aligned.

Extend the fingers and place all the fingertips together

9

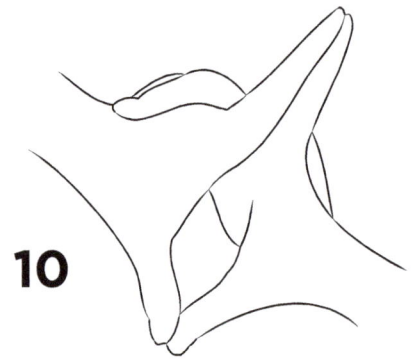

ENLIGHTENMENT
UTTARABODHI MUDRA

I am connected to my environment;
I am always searching for enlightenment.

Clasp hands together – extend pointer fingers up to touch together – and extend thumbs downward touching the tips together

10

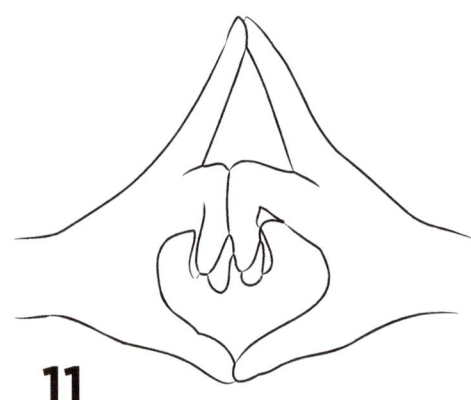

PATIENCE
KALESVANA MUDRA

I am patient – I am calm –
I now that time will carry on.

Touch the middle fingers together and touch the thumbs together- Bend the other fingers and touch the knuckles.

11

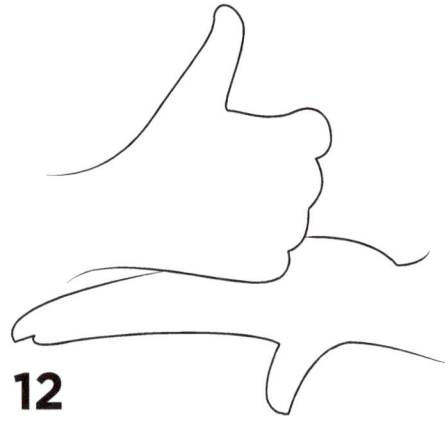

ENERGY CHANGING
SHIVALINA MUDRA

My perspective controls that way that I feel;
I can change my emotions and shift my ideals.

Place your right fist with thumb extended up into your left hand palm facing up.

12

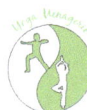

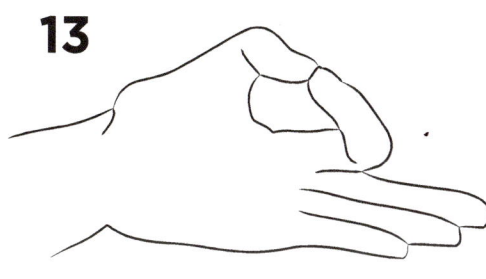

13

CONSCIOUSNESS
JNANA/GYAN/ INANA MUDRA

I am conscious of my thoughts and deeds;
I use my awareness to fulfill all my needs.

Touch the thumb and index fingers together – extend the other fingers and point the circle the fingers make upwards.

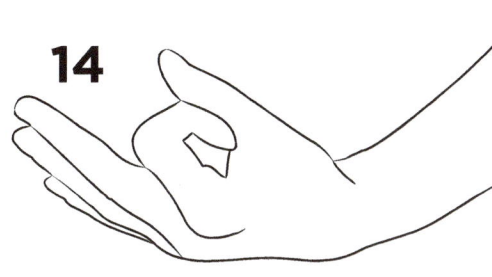

14

KNOWLEDGE
CHIN MUDRA

I am constantly learning something new;
Seeking knowledge and expanding what I can do.

Touch the thumb and index fingers together – extend the other fingers and point the circle the fingers make downward.

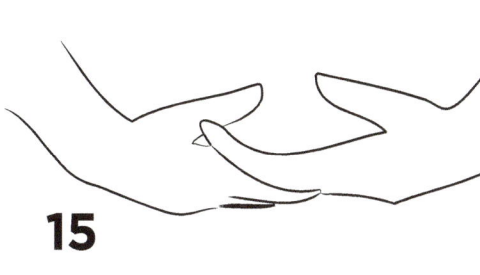

MEDITATION/CONTEMPLATION
DHYANI MUDRA

I take time to contemplate my thoughts;
Find my center and chart my course.

Place the left hand under the right hand with palms up and touch thumbs together.

15

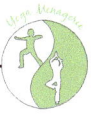

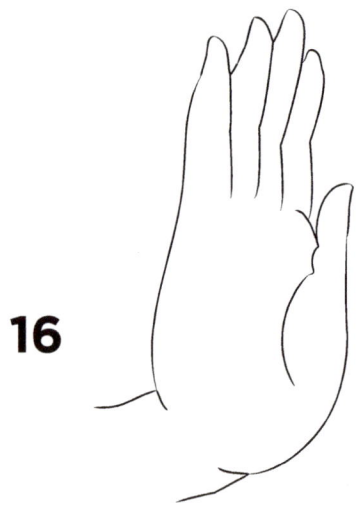

PROTECTION
ABHAYA MUDRA

I am safe – I am protected;
I am secure – I am connected.

Raise your right hand at chest level with palm facing forward, place the left hand on your thigh, lap or heart.

16

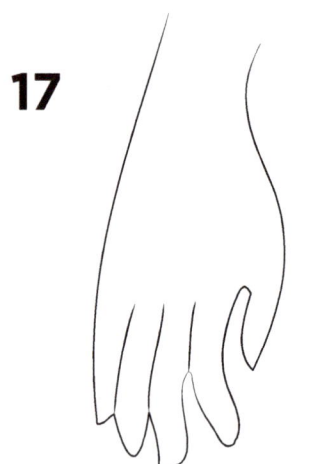

17

SEEKING WISDOM AND ENLIGHTENMENT
BHUMISPARSHA MUDRA

I am connected with everything;
I am content in my own being.

Point the left hand down toward the earth and let the fingertips touch the ground, Place the right hand palm up on your knee

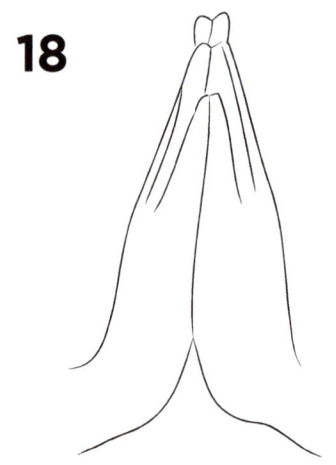

18

PRAYER
ATMANJALI MUDRA

I am thankful for everything;
I appreciate anything.

Place both hands together – fingertips pointing up

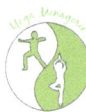

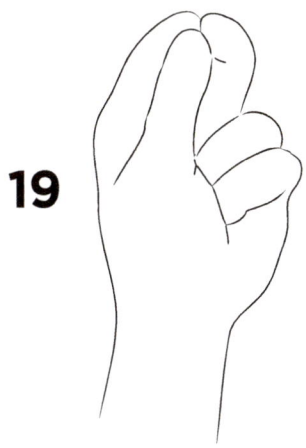

PROSPERITY
KUBERA MUDRA

I obtain all my goals;
I am prosperous in all my roles.

Touch the fingertips of your thumb, index and middle fingers together – curl the other fingers in the center of the palm

19

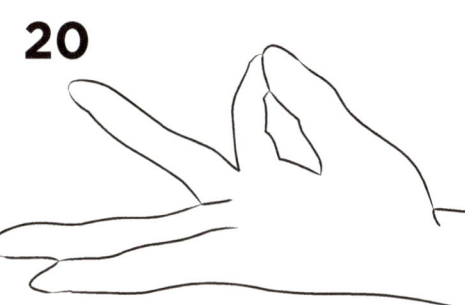

GOING WITH THE FLOW
BHUDI MUDRA

I am pure, I am refreshed;
I know that I am truly blessed.

Touch the tips of the thumb and pinky finger together-extend the other fingers

20

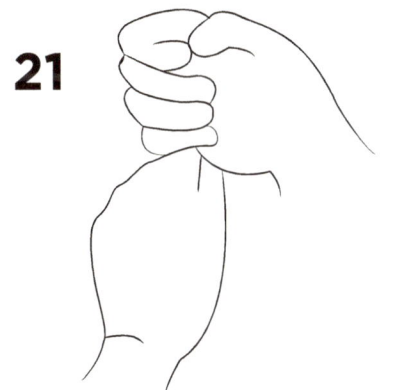

INNER SELF – SPIRIT
KUNDALINI MUDRA

I am grounded in my inner self;
I am centered and content with myself.

Create 2 fists (right on top) extend left index finger into the right fist

21

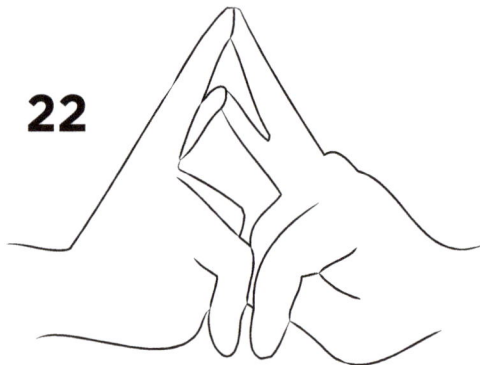

22

SELF
SHAKTI MUDRA

I open myself up and let my true self shine;
My thoughts and my feelings are authentically mine.

*Touch the fingertips of the pinky and ring fingers together –
bend the other fingers over the thumbs*

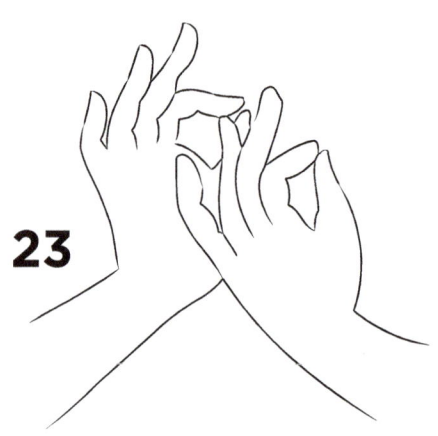

23

TURNING THE WHEEL
DHARMACHAKRA MUDRA

I am constantly moving like a turning wheel;
Changing, transforming and becoming real.

*Place the thumb and index fingers together on each hand,
left palm faces your heart, right palm faces outwards, touch
the middle finger of the left hand to the circle on the right
hand*

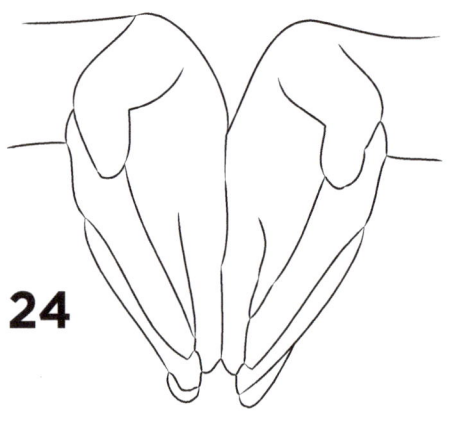

24

HANDFUL OF FLOWERS
PUSHPAPUTA MUDRA

With open hands and an open heart;
I open my mind and accept a new start.

*Place hands palms up touching pinky fingers and the side of
the hands together*

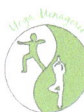

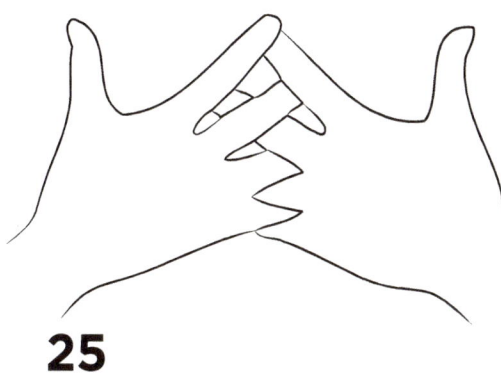

TRUST
VAJRAPRADAMA MUDRA

I trust in myself – I believe in me;
I am confident in my abilities.

Extend fingers and cross them in front of your chest

25

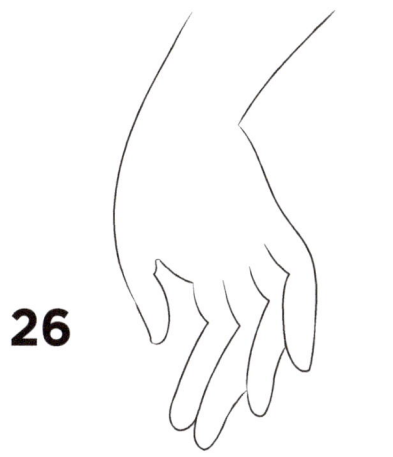

GRANTING WISHES OR MERCY
VARADA MUDRA

I am forgiving – I am fair;
I show mercy – I always share.

Left hand pam up pointed downward, Right hand on lap or thigh

26

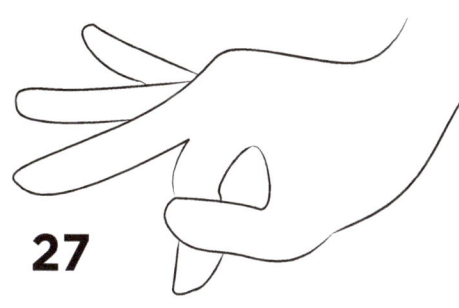

CONFIDENCE
AHAMKARA MUDRA

I am confident in what I can do;
To myself I am always true.

Touch the thumb to the 1st knuckle of the index finger and extend the other fingers

27

BALANCING
MAHASIRS MUDRA

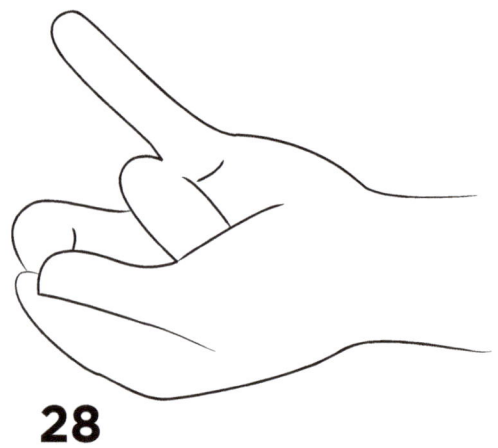

I am balanced and I am stable;
I am steady and I am able.

Touch the tips of the thumb, index and middle fingers together, Place ring finger in the fold of the thumb and extend pinky

28

STRESS RELIEF
DWIMUKHAM MUDRA

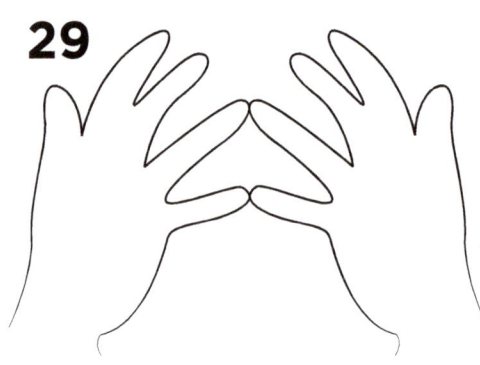

29

I release the stress from inside of me;
So I can live peacefully.

Hold the hands open with palms up and touch the tips of the ring and pinky fingers

CALMING
CHINMAYA MUDRA

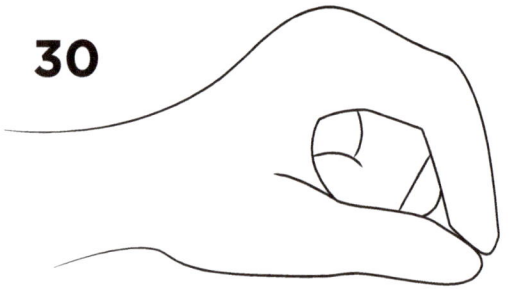

30

I am calm and have tranquility;
I am at peace with my reality.

Curl the middle, ring and pinky fingers, touch the tips of the index and thumbs together

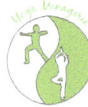

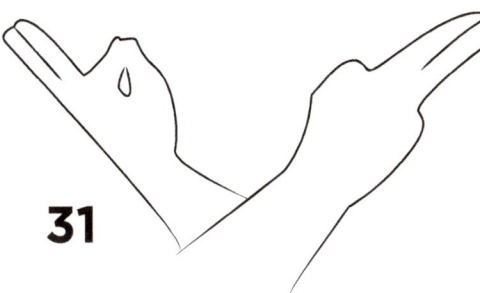

VICTORY
HUMKARA MUDRA

I am triumphant – I am victorious;
I am successful – I am glorious.

Cross the right forearm over the left forearm, touch the tips of the index and middle fingers with the thumb and extend the other fingers

31

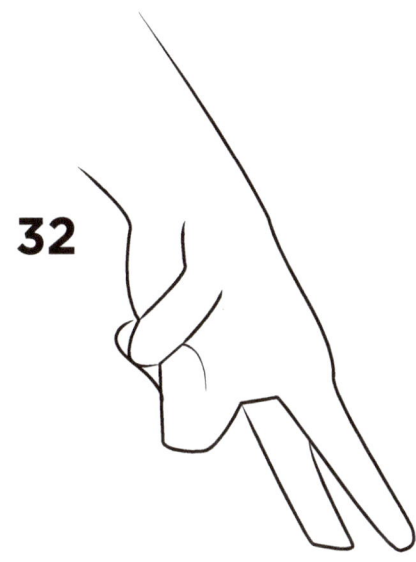

PEACE
BHU MUDRA

Inner peace inspires me;
To live my life in harmony.

Curl the ring and pinky fingers into the palm and cover with the thumb, extend the other fingers in a 'v' shape

32

LOVE
PURNA MUDRA

I give love everyday;
And I receive love in every way.

Interlace fingers and create a heart shape by touching the tips of the thumbs together

33

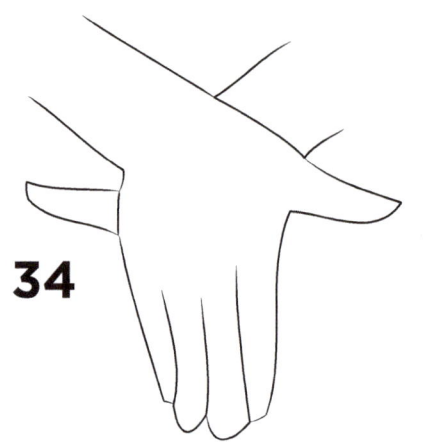

34

RELAXATION
MATSYA MUDRA

Every day I practice relaxation;
So I can feel peaceful sensations.

Place hands upon each other palms facing down and extend thumbs

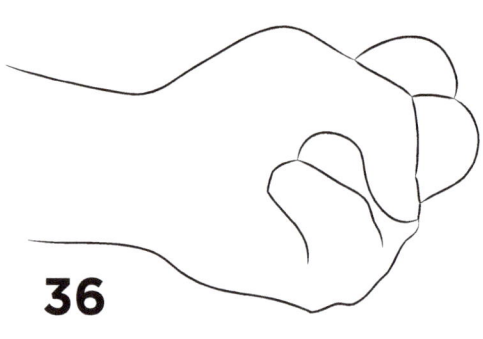

35

INNER STRENGTH
BRAHMA MUDRA

I gather up my inner strength;
I am willing to go to any length.

Make two fists with the hands and press the knuckles together

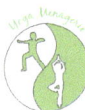

36

FIST/POWER
MUSHTI MUDRA

I believe in my strength and my inner power;
I am in control at every hour.

Curl the fingers inward, and cross the thumb over the ring finger

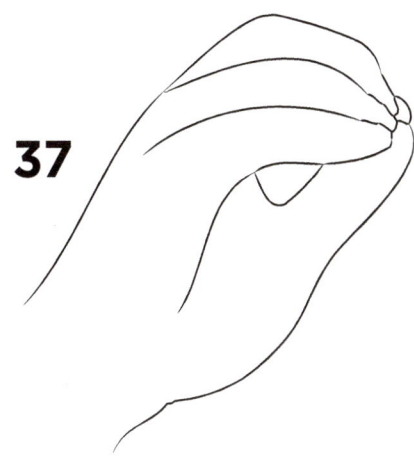

BEAK
MUKULA MUDRA

I empower myself – my strength comes from within–
I am ready for my healing to begin.

Place all four fingers on the thumbs and point towards any part of your body that needs healing or energy.

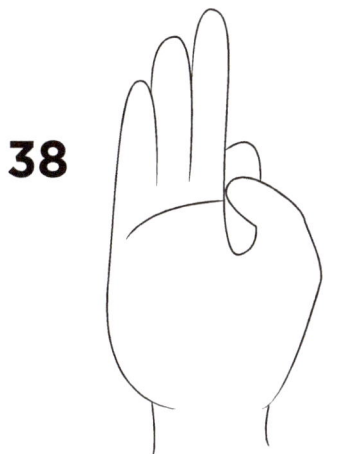

AIR/WIND
VAYU MUDRA

I am ever-changing like the breeze;
Following the flow with ease.

Bend the index finger down and cover with the thumb, extend the other fingers outward

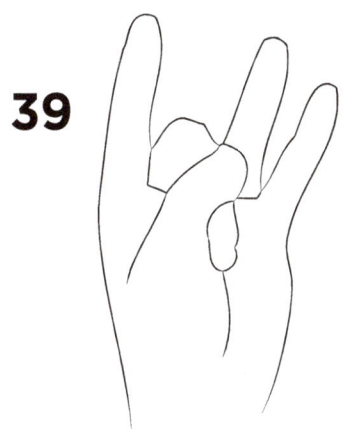

SKY / EMPTINESS
SHUNYA MUDRA

I open myself up and look to the sky;
I let my spirit free and fly.

Bend the middle finger down and cover with the thumb, extend the other fingers outward.

37

38

39

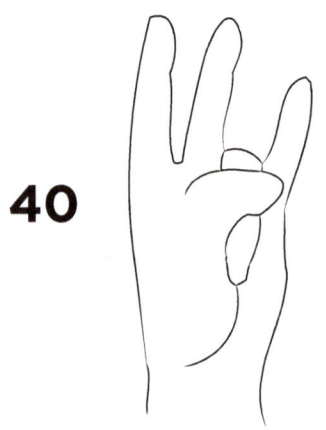

SUN
SURYA MUDRA

My inner light is as bright as the sun;
Shining down on everyone.

Curl the ring finger into the palm and cover with the thumb

40

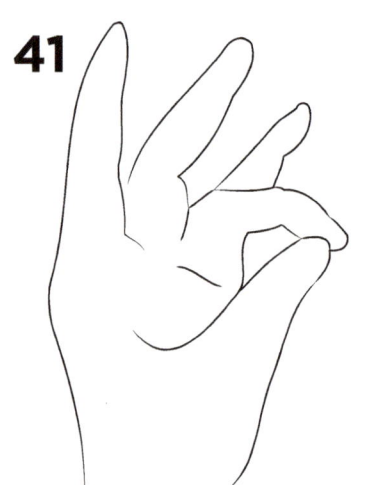

41

EARTH
PRITHIVI MUDRA

I am balanced and I am stable;
I am grounded and I am able.

Touch the thumb and ring finger together, extend the other fingers outward

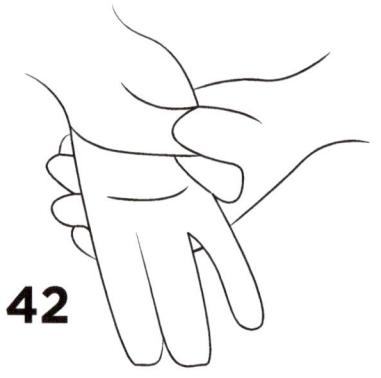

WATER
VARUNA MUDRA

I am like water nourishing and true;
Constantly changing but persistent too.

Right hand bend the pinky finger down, cover with thumb, circle that hand with the left.

42

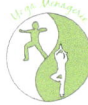

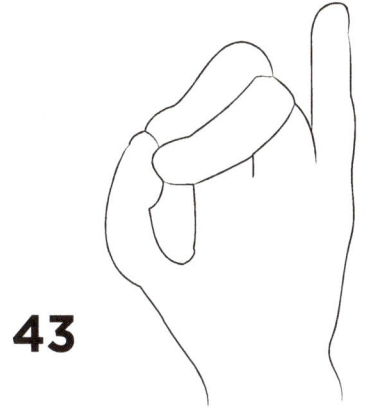

HEART
APAN VAYU MUDRA

I open my heart and let love free;
I allow my spirit to guide me.

Curl the index, middle and ring fingers into the palm, cover with the thumb and extend the pinky out

43

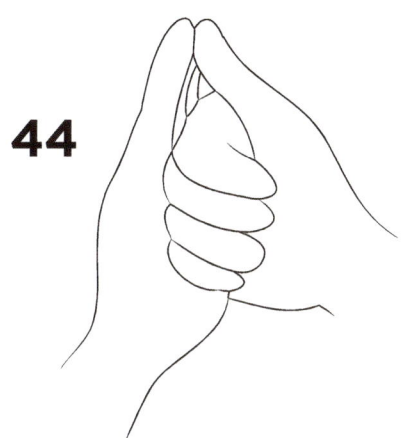

SHELL
SHANKH MUDRA

I listen to my inner voice;
My thoughts and my words are of my own choice.

Circle your left thumb with your right fingers and extend the right thumb to touch the extended fingers of the left hand

44

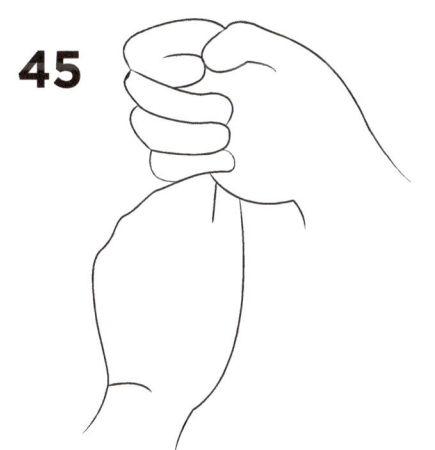

THUNDERBOLT
VAJRA MUDRA

I am like a thunderbolt – strong and bold;
I am ready to break the mold.

Extend the index finger and touch the other fingers to the thumb

45

BIRD
GARUDA MUDRA

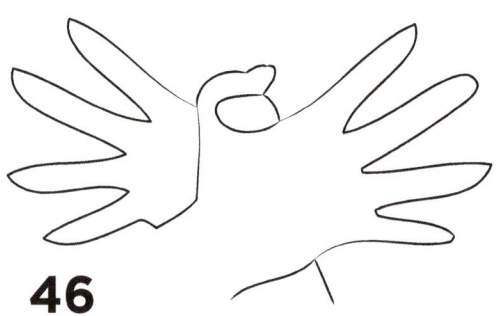

46

Just like a bird – I am free;
I soar to the places I want to be.

Cross thumbs together and extend the fingers

BEE
BHRAMARA MUDRA

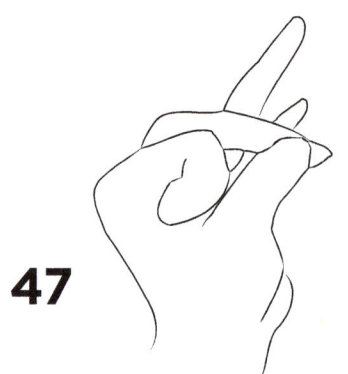

47

I work hard just like a bee;
I always give the best of me.

Curl the index finger into the thumb and touch the tips of the middle finger to the thumbs – extend the other fingers

ELEPHANT
GANESHA MUDRA

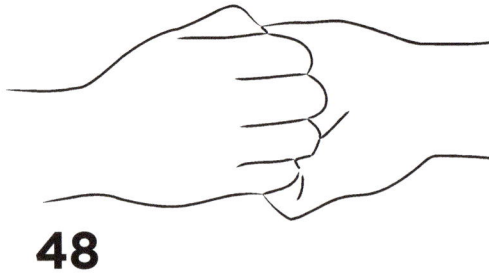

48

I have the strength of an elephant;
I can conquer the obstacles in my element.

Clasp all the fingers together – one palm faces front and the other back

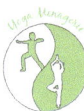

CROCODILE
MAKARA MUDRA

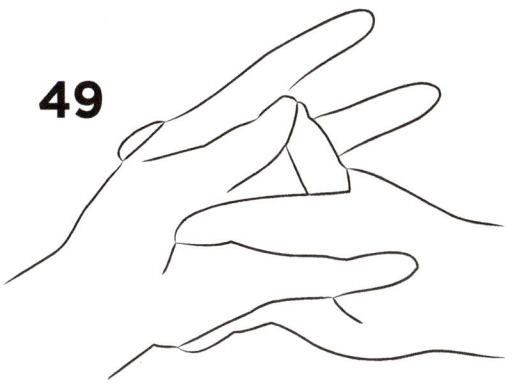

49

I am patient like a crocodile;
Observing the stillness is always worthwhile.

Extend one thumb to pinky and ring finger of the other hand, the other thumb touches the ring finger of the opposite hand.

SNAKE/STRENGTH AND WISDOM
NAGA MUDRA

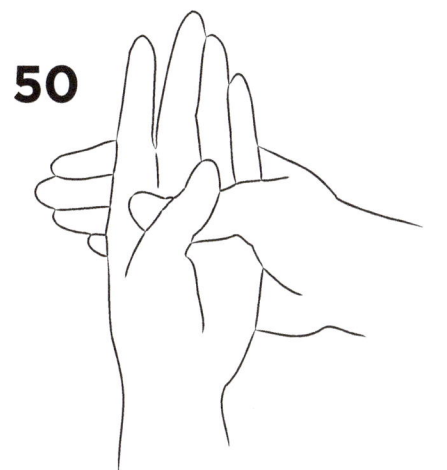

50

I respect the deepest insights from within me;
I open my mind and set myself free.

Cross your hands and your thumbs

About the Author

Con reprehe ndellore exerspi enimolupta sanimo dolorerate accum diti unt rehenet erro mos et explitisque se erit lique rest repro digenderum vercimus ea volupta tinctiam quis ereptus molum invererrupta nus aliscii scidita diosseque quis idunti asitia volupta tibus, nusam lab in porepel estibus.

Eriae maio. Occabor ad magnihi lloritae pa voluptis aut quia doluptae se nus vent verrovidel illessi molentiuntem vel in reped mostis si re eium quid unt ea voluptae lati asinvelendit vent lab il maios eume nobit quiatiur, volori omnis evenditas doluptur, que eos eumquatem fugit lant unt vella sincto eum, voluptatur, que eici restota speribus voloribus vitatem laboraeste et aliquam eius magnat il magnime et modit asperias sa dolorrum estia nonsedi utem non nist eum quam quam quuntius, ute sed qui torro temquat quamus.

Ecab il in necae reptur, quos quis dolenis aut fugit fugitent lit es molorestium nobit et est vernat hil int.

Quid magnate mporepu daectem quatibus delia il ium, con recum, consequist, que doluptiates voluptatate elique qui dis ilibus dolor aut veliqui aut etusciis debit quam core provid enimagnam fugiatis preprepre plicae niminul litios aut quam, audandi scipist, quos aliam erum restium senis et, si dolorio idio tet, officil magnima gnimet harchit ecaborum vendel inctenem dolorem unt vid qui te esequod quos apero que dolorerchil ipiciet volupta vellesti tem hil ipsa volorrovit que vid maxima voluptis quid ut aut odicid mo occumqui conseque nis iur? Sae quossun discimincia sa solor mod ea dusae pelit, tem untur?

Bit erspero vitemodi consed qui dolorerum in perunt.

Aperepero conessincia que es nis ipsumquatem nos dolorerspel int mosa venientiat assumquo occat enim facea nimaiorempos anda con natet et aut quos aut officium, quam

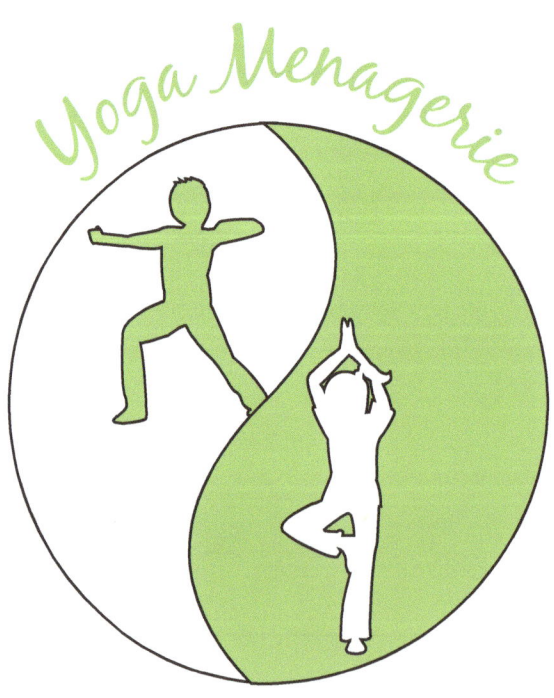